(GUIDE FOR USERS)

EMERGENCY CONTRACEPTION WITH POSTINOR

PREVENTING CONCEPTION USING THE MORNING-AFTER PILL

NICHOLE SCHEAFER

TABLE OF CONTENTS

CHAPTER ONE

INTRODUCTION TO EMERGENCY CONTRACEPTION

A. Understanding Emergency Contraception

Emergency contraception (EC) is a crucial aspect of reproductive healthcare, providing individuals with a safe and effective option to prevent unintended pregnancy after unprotected intercourse or contraceptive failure. Unlike regular forms of contraception, such as birth control pills or condoms, emergency contraception is specifically designed for use in emergencies and is intended to be used as soon as possible after unprotected sex.

Emergency contraception methods work by either preventing ovulation, fertilization, or implantation of a fertilized egg in the uterus. This helps to reduce the risk of pregnancy when regular contraception methods have failed or were not used. It's important to note that emergency contraception is not intended for routine use and should not replace regular contraceptive methods.

B. Importance of Timely Intervention

The effectiveness of emergency contraception is closely tied to the timing of its administration. In general, emergency contraception is most effective when taken as soon as possible after unprotected intercourse. As time passes, the likelihood of pregnancy increases, highlighting the importance of timely intervention.

For example, one of the most widely used forms of emergency contraception, levonorgestrel-based pills like Postinor 2, are most effective when taken within 24 hours of unprotected sex. While they can still provide some benefit up to 72 hours afterward, their efficacy decreases with each passing hour. Therefore, accessing emergency contraception promptly is critical for maximizing its effectiveness and reducing the risk of unintended pregnancy.

C. Overview of Postinor

Postinor 2, commonly known as the morning-after pill, is one of the most widely used forms of emergency contraception worldwide. It contains levonorgestrel, a synthetic hormone that is similar to the hormone progesterone, which is naturally produced by the ovaries. Levonorgestrel works primarily by inhibiting or delaying ovulation, thereby preventing the release of an egg for fertilization.

Postinor 2 is available in the form of oral tablets and is typically taken as a single dose. It can be purchased over-the-counter at pharmacies without a prescription in many countries, making it readily accessible for individuals in need of emergency contraception. However, it's important to note that the availability and accessibility of emergency contraception, including Postinor 2, may vary depending on local regulations and healthcare practices.

In addition to preventing ovulation, Postinor 2 may also alter cervical mucus and inhibit sperm transport, further reducing the likelihood of fertilization. It is important to understand that while emergency contraception like Postinor 2 can significantly reduce the risk of pregnancy, it is not 100% effective and should not be relied upon as a primary method of contraception.

Postinor 2 is generally well-tolerated, but like any medication, it may cause side effects in some individuals. Common side effects may include nausea, vomiting, abdominal pain, fatigue, and changes in menstrual bleeding patterns. These side effects are usually mild and temporary, resolving on their own within a few days. However, individuals who experience severe or persistent side effects should seek medical attention promptly.

CHAPTER TWO

HOW POSTINOR WORKS

A. Mechanism of Action

Postinor, also known as the morning-after pill or emergency contraception, primarily works by preventing ovulation, which is the release of an egg from the ovaries. The active ingredient in Postinor is levonorgestrel, a synthetic hormone that is similar to the hormone progesterone, which is naturally produced by the ovaries.

When taken as directed, Postinor inhibits or delays ovulation by altering the hormonal signals that regulate the menstrual cycle. By preventing ovulation, Postinor reduces the likelihood of an egg being released from the ovaries and therefore decreases the chances of fertilization occurring if unprotected intercourse has taken place.

In addition to preventing ovulation, Postinor may also affect other aspects of the reproductive process to further reduce the risk of pregnancy. For example, it may alter the consistency of cervical mucus, making it more difficult for sperm to reach the egg. Postinor may also affect the lining of the uterus, making it less receptive to implantation if fertilization does occur.

B. Effectiveness in Preventing Pregnancy

The effectiveness of Postinor in preventing pregnancy depends on several factors, including the timing of its administration and individual variations in response to the medication. When taken within the recommended time frame, Postinor can significantly reduce the risk of pregnancy after unprotected intercourse.

Studies have shown that Postinor is most effective when taken as soon as possible after unprotected sex, with efficacy rates highest within the first 24 hours. However, it can still provide some benefit when taken up to 72 hours (3 days) after intercourse. As time passes, the likelihood of pregnancy increases, so timely intervention is crucial for maximizing the effectiveness of Postinor.

While Postinor is highly effective at preventing pregnancy when used correctly, it is not 100% guaranteed, and there is still a small risk of contraceptive failure. It is important for individuals to understand that emergency contraception should not be relied upon as a regular form of birth control and that they should consider using a more reliable contraceptive method for ongoing protection against pregnancy.

C. Timing and Administration

The timing of Postinor administration is critical for maximizing its effectiveness in preventing pregnancy. Postinor should be taken as soon as possible after unprotected intercourse, ideally within the first 24 hours, to achieve the best results. However, it can still be effective when taken up to 72 hours after intercourse.

Postinor is available in the form of oral tablets, which are typically taken as a single dose. The tablet should be swallowed whole with water and can be taken with or without food. It is essential to follow the instructions provided with the medication carefully and to take the full dose as directed.

In addition to timing, individual factors such as body weight, medical history, and medication interactions may also influence the effectiveness of Postinor. While Postinor is generally well-tolerated, some individuals may experience side effects such as nausea, vomiting, abdominal pain, fatigue, or changes in menstrual bleeding patterns. These side effects are usually mild and temporary, resolving on their own within a few days.

CHAPTER THREE

INDICATIONS FOR POSTINOR USE

A. Situations Requiring Emergency Contraception

Emergency contraception becomes imperative in various scenarios where regular contraception methods fail or are absent. Firstly, instances of unprotected intercourse due to condom breakage or slippage, missed contraceptive pills, or incorrect usage of barrier methods warrant immediate attention. Moreover, sexual assault survivors may urgently require emergency contraception to prevent unwanted pregnancies resulting from non-consensual intercourse.

Furthermore, in cases where individuals forget to use contraception during their fertile window or engage in unplanned sexual activity without contraception, Postinor can serve as a vital recourse. Its timely use can avert the challenges and emotional toll associated with an unplanned pregnancy, empowering individuals to regain control over their reproductive choices.

B. Criteria for Postinor Consideration

While Postinor offers a valuable solution in emergencies, certain criteria must guide its consideration to ensure its appropriate and effective use. Firstly, the timeframe for administering Postinor is critical. It is most effective when taken within 72 hours (three days) after unprotected intercourse, although its efficacy diminishes over time. Therefore, prompt action is essential to maximize its effectiveness.

Additionally, individuals must consider their menstrual cycle phase when contemplating Postinor use. While it can be effective throughout the menstrual cycle, its efficacy may vary depending on the timing concerning ovulation. Counseling individuals to understand their menstrual cycle and the potential implications on emergency contraception can aid in informed decision-making.

Furthermore, individuals with contraindications to levonorgestrel, the active ingredient in Postinor, should seek alternative emergency contraception methods. Conditions such as severe liver disease, unexplained vaginal bleeding, or known hypersensitivity to levonorgestrel necessitate alternative approaches to prevent unwanted pregnancies.

C. Counseling Prior to Postinor Use

Effective counseling before Postinor use is crucial to ensure individuals make informed decisions aligned with their health needs and preferences. Firstly, healthcare providers must provide comprehensive information about emergency contraception, including its mechanism of action, efficacy rates, and potential side effects.

Moreover, counseling should address alternative emergency contraception methods, such as the copper intrauterine device (IUD), which offers a highly effective option for up to five days after unprotected intercourse. Providing individuals with a range of options empowers them to choose the most suitable method based on their individual circumstances and preferences.

Furthermore, counseling sessions should emphasize the temporary nature of emergency contraception and the importance of regular contraception for long-term pregnancy prevention. Encouraging individuals to explore and access regular contraceptive methods tailored to their needs can help prevent future contraceptive emergencies.

Importantly, counseling sessions should create a supportive and non-judgmental environment where individuals feel comfortable discussing their concerns, preferences, and any barriers to contraception use. Addressing potential stigma or misconceptions surrounding emergency contraception can foster open communication and facilitate informed decision-making.

Additionally, counseling should cover the importance of follow-up care, including pregnancy testing if menstruation is delayed by more than a week after taking Postinor. This ensures timely identification of any potential pregnancy and appropriate support and guidance for individuals navigating their reproductive health journey.

CHAPTER FOUR

DOSAGE AND ADMINISTRATION

A. Recommended Dosage Regimen

The recommended dosage regimen for Postinor typically involves taking a single tablet containing levonorgestrel, the active ingredient, as soon as possible after unprotected intercourse. Ideally, it should be administered within 72 hours (three days) of sexual activity to maximize its effectiveness in preventing pregnancy. However, it's crucial to note that the sooner it is taken after intercourse, the higher the likelihood of preventing pregnancy.

In some regions, emergency contraception may be available in two doses, with the second dose taken 12 hours after the first. This regimen, known as the Yuzpe regimen, involves taking two tablets containing levonorgestrel within a specified timeframe to achieve optimal efficacy. However, the single-dose regimen is more commonly recommended due to its simplicity and comparable effectiveness.

B. Guidelines for Taking Postinor

Proper administration of Postinor is essential to ensure its efficacy in preventing pregnancy and minimize the risk of adverse effects. Individuals should follow these guidelines when taking Postinor:

Timing: Take the tablet(s) as soon as possible after unprotected intercourse, ideally within 72 hours (three days) for optimal effectiveness. Delaying administration reduces its efficacy in preventing pregnancy.

Administration: Swallow the tablet(s) whole with water. Do not chew or crush them, as this may affect the absorption of the medication.

Food: Postinor can be taken with or without food. However, if it causes stomach upset, taking it with a meal or snack may help alleviate discomfort.

Avoiding Vomiting: If vomiting occurs within two hours of taking Postinor, it may affect its absorption and efficacy. In such cases, individuals should contact a healthcare provider for further guidance and possible re-administration of the medication.

Regular Contraception: Postinor is intended for emergency use only and should not replace regular contraceptive methods. Individuals should continue or initiate a regular contraceptive method to prevent future unplanned pregnancies.

Follow-up Care: It's important to follow up with a healthcare provider if menstruation is delayed by more than a week after taking Postinor or if there are any concerns about potential pregnancy. Pregnancy testing and further evaluation may be necessary to ensure appropriate care and support.

C. Considerations for Repeat Use

While Postinor is designed for emergency use, some individuals may find themselves requiring emergency contraception on multiple occasions. In such cases, several considerations come into play:

Frequency: Postinor is intended for occasional and emergency use only. Repeat use within the same menstrual cycle or frequent reliance on emergency contraception can disrupt menstrual patterns and increase the risk of side effects.

Alternative Options: Individuals who require emergency contraception on a recurrent basis should explore alternative contraceptive options, such as long-acting reversible contraceptives (LARCs) like intrauterine devices (IUDs) or contraceptive implants. These methods offer highly effective, long-term contraception without the need for repeated emergency interventions.

Health Monitoring: Healthcare providers should monitor individuals who require repeat use of emergency contraception for any potential health implications, such as changes in menstrual patterns, hormonal imbalances, or side effects associated with frequent use of levonorgestrel-containing medications.

Counseling and Support: Repeat users of emergency contraception may benefit from additional counseling and support to address underlying contraceptive needs, barriers to regular contraception use, and strategies for preventing future unplanned pregnancies. Providing comprehensive reproductive healthcare and support services can empower individuals to make informed decisions about their contraceptive choices and overall reproductive health.

CHAPTER FIVE

POTENTIAL SIDE EFFECTS

A. Common Side Effects

While many individuals tolerate Postinor 2 well, some may experience common side effects that typically resolve on their own without medical intervention. These side effects may include:

Nausea and Vomiting: Nausea is one of the most frequently reported side effects of Postinor 2. Some individuals may also experience vomiting, particularly if the medication is taken on an empty stomach. Taking the pill with food or a snack may help alleviate these symptoms.

Fatigue: Feelings of tiredness or fatigue are common after taking Postinor 2. These symptoms usually subside within a few days.

Headache: Headaches or migraines may occur as a result of hormonal changes induced by the medication. Over-the-counter pain relievers and rest can help alleviate discomfort.

Abdominal Pain or Cramping: Some individuals may experience abdominal discomfort or cramping after taking Postinor

2. This is typically mild and resolves on its own.

Changes in Menstrual Cycle: Postinor 2 may temporarily alter the menstrual cycle, leading to irregular bleeding or changes in menstrual flow. These changes are usually temporary and should normalize within a few weeks.

It's important to note that experiencing these side effects does not necessarily indicate a complication or failure of the medication. Most individuals tolerate Postinor 2 well, and these side effects are generally mild and transient.

B. Rare but Serious Adverse Reactions

While uncommon, Postinor 2 may rarely cause serious adverse reactions that require medical attention. These include:

Allergic Reactions: In rare cases, individuals may experience allergic reactions to the medication, characterized by symptoms such as rash, itching, swelling of the face or throat, and difficulty breathing. Allergic reactions require immediate medical attention.

Ectopic Pregnancy: Although extremely rare, there have been reports of ectopic pregnancy (pregnancy outside the uterus) following the use of emergency contraception. Individuals experiencing severe abdominal pain, shoulder pain, or fainting after taking Postinor 2 should seek immediate medical attention, as these may be signs of an ectopic pregnancy.

Severe Abdominal Pain: While mild abdominal discomfort is common after taking Postinor 2, severe or persistent abdominal pain may indicate a more serious underlying condition, such as ovarian cyst rupture or appendicitis. Individuals experiencing severe abdominal pain should seek medical evaluation promptly.

Menstrual Irregularities: While changes in the menstrual cycle are expected after taking Postinor 2, persistent or severe menstrual irregularities may require further evaluation by a healthcare provider to rule out underlying causes.

It's important for individuals to be aware of these rare but serious adverse reactions and seek medical attention if they experience any concerning symptoms after taking Postinor 2.

C. Management of Side Effects

Effective management of side effects associated with Postinor 2 involves both self-care measures and, in some cases, medical intervention. Some strategies for managing common side effects include:

Nausea and Vomiting: Taking the pill with food or a snack can help reduce the likelihood of nausea and vomiting. Over-the-counter anti-nausea medications may also provide relief.

Headache: Rest, hydration, and over-the-counter pain relievers such as ibuprofen or acetaminophen can help alleviate headache symptoms.

Abdominal Pain or Cramping: Applying a heating pad to the abdomen or taking over-the-counter pain relievers can help relieve abdominal discomfort.

Fatigue: Ensuring adequate rest and hydration can help alleviate feelings of tiredness or fatigue.

In cases of rare but serious adverse reactions, such as allergic reactions or severe abdominal pain, individuals should seek immediate medical attention. Healthcare providers can assess the severity of symptoms, provide appropriate treatment, and ensure individuals receive the care they need.

CHAPTER SIX

SAFETY AND CONTRAINDICATIONS

A. Precautions for Postinor Use

While Postinor 2 is generally safe and well-tolerated, certain precautions should be observed to maximize its effectiveness and minimize potential risks. These precautions include:

Timing of Administration: Postinor 2 should be taken as soon as possible after unprotected intercourse, ideally within 72 hours (three days) for optimal efficacy. Delaying administration beyond this timeframe reduces its effectiveness in preventing pregnancy.

Regular Contraception: Postinor 2 is intended for emergency use only and should not replace regular contraceptive methods. Individuals should continue or initiate a regular contraceptive method to prevent future unplanned pregnancies.

Follow-up Care: It's important to follow up with a healthcare provider if menstruation is delayed by more than a week after taking Postinor 2 or if there are any concerns about potential pregnancy. Pregnancy testing and further evaluation may be necessary to ensure appropriate care and support.

Avoiding Repeated Use: Postinor 2 should not be used as a regular form of contraception. Repeated or frequent use of emergency contraception can disrupt menstrual patterns and increase the risk of side effects. Individuals requiring frequent emergency contraception should explore alternative contraceptive options.

B. Medical Conditions Requiring Caution

Certain medical conditions may require caution or closer monitoring when considering the use of Postinor 2. These conditions include:

Liver Disease: Individuals with severe liver disease may be at increased risk of adverse effects from Postinor 2, as the medication is metabolized in the liver. Close monitoring and consideration of alternative contraceptive options may be necessary in these cases.

Unexplained Vaginal Bleeding: Postinor 2 may exacerbate unexplained vaginal bleeding, and its use should be avoided in individuals experiencing abnormal or persistent vaginal bleeding until the underlying cause is diagnosed and addressed.

Hypersensitivity to Levonorgestrel: Individuals with a known hypersensitivity or allergy to levonorgestrel, the active ingredient in Postinor 2, should avoid its use and explore alternative emergency contraception options.

Breast Cancer: While the evidence is limited, some studies suggest a potential association between hormonal contraceptives containing progestogens like levonorgestrel and an increased risk of breast cancer. Individuals with a history of breast cancer or other estrogen-sensitive tumors should discuss the risks and benefits of Postinor 2 with their healthcare provider.

C. Interactions with Other Medications

Postinor 2 may interact with certain medications, potentially affecting its efficacy or increasing the risk of adverse effects. These interactions include:

Enzyme Inducers: Drugs that induce hepatic enzymes, such as certain anticonvulsants (e.g., phenytoin, carbamazepine) and rifampicin, may accelerate the metabolism of levonorgestrel, reducing its effectiveness. Alternative contraceptive methods should be considered in individuals taking enzyme-inducing medications.

Antibiotics: While the evidence is inconclusive, some antibiotics may theoretically reduce the effectiveness of hormonal contraceptives like Postinor 2 by altering gut flora and impairing enterohepatic circulation. Additional contraceptive precautions, such as barrier methods, may be advisable during antibiotic therapy.

Herbal Supplements: Certain herbal supplements, such as St. John's wort, may induce hepatic enzymes and potentially reduce the effectiveness of hormonal contraceptives. Individuals should consult their healthcare provider before combining herbal supplements with Postinor 2.

HIV Medications: Some antiretroviral medications used in the treatment of HIV/AIDS may interact with hormonal contraceptives, potentially affecting their efficacy. Close monitoring and consideration of alternative contraceptive methods may be necessary in individuals receiving HIV treatment.

CHAPTER SEVEN

EFFECTIVENESS AND FOLLOW-UP

Postinor 2 stands as a crucial pillar in the realm of emergency contraception, offering individuals a timely recourse to prevent unplanned pregnancies. Understanding its effectiveness rates, the importance of follow-up care, and options for ongoing contraceptive needs is paramount in ensuring individuals receive comprehensive reproductive healthcare.

A. Postinor Efficacy Rates

The efficacy of Postinor 2 in preventing pregnancy depends on several factors, including the timing of administration and individual characteristics. When taken within 72 hours (three days) of unprotected intercourse, Postinor 2 is estimated to prevent approximately 75-89% of pregnancies. However, its efficacy decreases with time, emphasizing the importance of prompt administration.

It's crucial to note that emergency contraception, including Postinor 2, is not 100% effective and should not be relied upon as a primary contraceptive method. Despite its high efficacy when used correctly, there is still a risk of pregnancy, particularly if taken after the optimal timeframe or in cases of repeated use.

B. Importance of Follow-Up Care

While Postinor 2 offers a valuable option for emergency contraception, follow-up care is essential to ensure individuals receive appropriate support and guidance. Follow-up care serves several important purposes:

Pregnancy Testing: Individuals should follow up with a healthcare provider if menstruation is delayed by more than a week after taking Postinor 2. Pregnancy testing can help rule out pregnancy and provide reassurance or prompt further evaluation and care if necessary.

Addressing Concerns: Follow-up appointments provide an opportunity for individuals to address any concerns or questions they may have about emergency contraception, potential side effects, or ongoing contraceptive needs. Healthcare providers can offer guidance and support tailored to each individual's circumstances and preferences.

Discussing Ongoing Contraceptive Needs: Follow-up appointments also offer an opportunity to discuss ongoing contraceptive needs and explore options for long-term contraception. Individuals can receive information about various contraceptive methods, their efficacy, and suitability based on factors such as medical history, lifestyle, and preferences.

Monitoring Side Effects: Some individuals may experience side effects or adverse reactions after taking Postinor 2. Follow-up care allows healthcare providers to monitor these symptoms, provide appropriate management, and ensure individuals receive the care they need.

Preventing Future Unplanned Pregnancies: By discussing ongoing contraceptive needs and providing access to effective contraception, follow-up care helps prevent future unplanned pregnancies and promotes individuals' overall reproductive health and well-being.

C. Options for Ongoing Contraceptive Needs

Following emergency contraception with Postinor 2, individuals should explore options for ongoing contraceptive needs to prevent future unplanned pregnancies. Several contraceptive methods are available, each with its own benefits, efficacy rates, and considerations:

Barrier Methods: Condoms, both male and female, offer protection against both pregnancy and sexually transmitted infections (STIs). They are readily available, easy to use, and do not require a prescription.

Hormonal Contraceptives: Birth control pills, patches, injections, and vaginal rings contain hormones that prevent ovulation and/or thicken cervical mucus, thereby preventing pregnancy. These methods offer high efficacy when used correctly and consistently.

Long-Acting Reversible Contraceptives (LARCs): Intrauterine devices (IUDs) and contraceptive implants provide highly effective, long-term contraception without the need for daily adherence. They are suitable for individuals seeking reliable contraception for several years.

Sterilization: Permanent methods of contraception, such as tubal ligation or vasectomy, offer a highly effective option for individuals who have completed their desired family size and wish to permanently prevent pregnancy.

Natural Family Planning: Some individuals may opt for natural family planning methods, such as fertility awareness-based methods (FABMs), which involve tracking menstrual cycles and avoiding intercourse during fertile periods. While less effective than other methods, FABMs can be a suitable option for individuals with religious or personal objections to hormonal contraception.

It's essential for individuals to discuss their contraceptive options with a healthcare provider to determine the most suitable method based on their individual needs, preferences, and medical history. By exploring ongoing contraceptive needs and accessing appropriate methods, individuals can take proactive steps to prevent future unplanned pregnancies and promote their reproductive health and well-being.

CHAPTER EIGHT

ADDRESSING MISCONCEPTIONS

A. Clarifying Myths and Dispelling Misinformation

First and foremost, one prevalent myth surrounding Postinor 2 is its efficacy. Some individuals mistakenly believe that taking the morning-after pill guarantees 100% protection against pregnancy. However, this is far from the truth. Postinor 2 is designed to reduce the risk of pregnancy after unprotected intercourse, but it is not foolproof. Its effectiveness diminishes over time, with the highest efficacy when taken within the first 24 hours and decreasing thereafter. Additionally, it may not prevent pregnancy in every instance, especially if ovulation has already occurred. Therefore, while Postinor 2 is a valuable option for emergency contraception, it should not be considered a substitute for regular birth control methods.

Dispelling another common misconception, there's a belief that frequent use of Postinor 2 is harmless. Some individuals may rely on it as their primary method of contraception, assuming that its occasional use won't pose any risks. However, frequent use of emergency contraception can disrupt hormonal balance and menstrual cycles, leading to irregular periods and other complications. Moreover, it's important to remember that Postinor 2 is not intended for regular use and should only be used as a backup in emergency situations.

Furthermore, there are concerns about the safety of Postinor 2 and its potential side effects. While like any medication, it can cause side effects in some individuals, the majority of users tolerate it well. Common side effects may include nausea, vomiting, fatigue, breast tenderness, and changes in menstrual bleeding patterns. However, these side effects are usually mild and transient, resolving within a few days. Serious complications from Postinor 2 are rare, but individuals with certain medical conditions, such as liver disease or a history of blood clots, should consult a healthcare provider before using it.

Addressing the misconception that emergency contraception promotes promiscuity is also essential. Some critics argue that easy access to emergency contraception encourages risky sexual behavior and undermines personal responsibility. However, research indicates that increased availability of emergency contraception does not lead to an increase in sexual activity or unprotected intercourse. Instead, it provides individuals with a crucial option to prevent unintended pregnancies when other methods fail or are unavailable. Moreover, promoting access to emergency contraception aligns with public health goals of reducing the number of unplanned pregnancies and improving maternal and child health outcomes.

Another misconception worth addressing is the belief that emergency contraception is equivalent to abortion. This misconception stems from a misunderstanding of how emergency contraception works. Postinor 2 primarily works by delaying or inhibiting ovulation, thereby preventing fertilization. It may also affect the cervical mucus and uterine lining, making it difficult for sperm to reach the egg or for a fertilized egg to implant in the uterus. However, it does not terminate an established pregnancy. Emergency contraception should be taken as soon as possible after unprotected intercourse to maximize its effectiveness in preventing pregnancy.

Education plays a pivotal role in dispelling myths and misconceptions surrounding Postinor 2 and other contraceptive methods. Providing accurate information about how emergency contraception works, its effectiveness, potential side effects, and appropriate usage can empower individuals to make informed decisions about their reproductive health. Healthcare providers, educators, and community organizations have a responsibility to offer comprehensive and nonjudgmental guidance on contraceptive options, including emergency contraception.

CHAPTER NINE

CONCLUSION

Firstly, it's essential to understand the role and limitations of emergency contraception. Postinor 2, commonly referred to as the morning-after pill, is not a regular contraceptive method. Instead, it serves as a backup option to prevent pregnancy after unprotected intercourse or contraceptive failure. However, its effectiveness diminishes over time, emphasizing the importance of prompt usage.

Recapping key points, we must address prevalent misconceptions surrounding Postinor 2. It does not guarantee 100% protection against pregnancy, nor is it intended for frequent use. Understanding its mechanism of action—primarily delaying or inhibiting ovulation—dispels misconceptions equating it to abortion. Furthermore, while it's generally safe, like any medication, it can cause side effects, though severe complications are rare.

Encouraging informed decision-making is paramount in navigating reproductive health choices. Individuals must be empowered with accurate information about emergency contraception, including its efficacy, usage guidelines, and potential side effects. This empowerment fosters autonomy, enabling individuals to make choices aligned with their values and circumstances.

Advocating for accessible reproductive healthcare is crucial in ensuring equitable access to emergency contraception and comprehensive contraceptive services. Access barriers such as cost, stigma, and limited availability disproportionately affect marginalized communities, hindering their ability to make informed choices about their reproductive health. By advocating for policies that promote affordability, destigmatization, and widespread availability of emergency contraception, we can contribute to reproductive justice for all.

Moreover, comprehensive sex education plays a pivotal role in promoting informed decision-making and reducing unintended pregnancies. By providing accurate information about contraception, including emergency contraception, educators can empower individuals to make responsible choices regarding their sexual health. Additionally, destigmatizing discussions about emergency contraception fosters open communication, reducing shame and promoting access to necessary resources.

FINALLY, navigating emergency contraception with Postinor 2 requires a nuanced understanding of its role, limitations, and implications. By recapping key points, encouraging informed decision-making, and advocating for accessible reproductive healthcare, we can empower individuals to make choices aligned with their reproductive goals and values. Together, let's strive for a world where everyone has equitable access to comprehensive reproductive healthcare and the agency to make informed decisions about their bodies and futures.